This Book Belongs to

_____

_____

_____

In case of emergency

Name: _____

Phone:_____

Email: _____

Address:_____

_____

	Calories	Carbs (g)	Sugars (g)	Fiber (g)	Protein (g)	Fat (g)
Date: _____						
Weight: _____						
Daily Goal: _____						
Breakfast: Time:						
Lunch: Time:						
Dinner: Time:						
Page Totals:						

		Calories	Carbs (g)	Sugars (g)	Fiber (g)	Protein (g)	Fat (g)
Sleep: _____							
Water: _____							
Mood: _____							
Other Meals / Snacks:							
Page Totals:							

Blood Sugar Log:	Before	After	Insulin	Meds
Breakfast				
Lunch				
Dinner				

Activity - Exercise:	Duration	Calories	Intensity

Other Notes, Vitamins, Supplements Meds:

_____

_____

_____

_____

	Calories	Carbs (g)	Sugars (g)	Fiber (g)	Protein (g)	Fat (g)
Date: _____						
Weight: _____						
Daily Goal: _____						
Breakfast: Time:						
Lunch: Time:						
Dinner: Time:						
Page Totals:						

	Calories	Carbs (g)	Sugars (g)	Fiber (g)	Protein (g)	Fat (g)
Sleep: _____ Water: _____ Mood: _____						

Other Meals / Snacks:						
Page Totals:						

Blood Sugar Log:	Before	After	Insulin	Meds
Breakfast				
Lunch				
Dinner				

Activity - Exercise:	Duration	Calories	Intensity

Other Notes, Vitamins, Supplements Meds:

_____

_____

_____

_____

	Calories	Carbs (g)	Sugars (g)	Fiber (g)	Protein (g)	Fat (g)
Date: _____						
Weight: _____						
Daily Goal: _____						
Breakfast: Time:						
Lunch: Time:						
Dinner: Time:						
Page Totals:						

		Calories	Carbs (g)	Sugars (g)	Fiber (g)	Protein (g)	Fat (g)
Sleep: _____							
Water: _____							
Mood: _____							
Other Meals / Snacks:							
Page Totals:							

Blood Sugar Log:	Before	After	Insulin	Meds
Breakfast				
Lunch				
Dinner				

Activity - Exercise:	Duration	Calories	Intensity

Other Notes, Vitamins, Supplements Meds:

_____

_____

_____

_____

	Calories	Carbs (g)	Sugars (g)	Fiber (g)	Protein (g)	Fat (g)
Date: _____						
Weight: _____						
Daily Goal: _____						
Breakfast: Time:						
Lunch: Time:						
Dinner: Time:						
Page Totals:						

	Calories	Carbs (g)	Sugars (g)	Fiber (g)	Protein (g)	Fat (g)
Sleep: _____ Water: _____ Mood: _____						
Other Meals / Snacks:						
Page Totals:						

Blood Sugar Log:	Before	After	Insulin	Meds
Breakfast				
Lunch				
Dinner				

Activity - Exercise:	Duration	Calories	Intensity

Other Notes, Vitamins, Supplements Meds:

_____

_____

_____

_____

	Calories	Carbs (g)	Sugars (g)	Fiber (g)	Protein (g)	Fat (g)
Date:						
Weight:						
Daily Goal:						
Breakfast: Time:						
Lunch: Time:						
Dinner: Time:						
Page Totals:						

	Calories	Carbs (g)	Sugars (g)	Fiber (g)	Protein (g)	Fat (g)
Sleep: _____						
Water: _____						
Mood: _____						
Other Meals / Snacks:						
Page Totals:						

Blood Sugar Log:	Before	After	Insulin	Meds
Breakfast				
Lunch				
Dinner				

Activity - Exercise:	Duration	Calories	Intensity

Other Notes, Vitamins, Supplements Meds:

_____

_____

_____

_____

	Calories	Carbs (g)	Sugars (g)	Fiber (g)	Protein (g)	Fat (g)
Date: _____						
Weight: _____						
Daily Goal: _____						
Breakfast: Time:						
Lunch: Time:						
Dinner: Time:						
Page Totals:						

	Calories	Carbs (g)	Sugars (g)	Fiber (g)	Protein (g)	Fat (g)
Sleep: _____ Water: _____ Mood: _____						
Other Meals / Snacks:						
Page Totals:						

Blood Sugar Log:	Before	After	Insulin	Meds
Breakfast				
Lunch				
Dinner				

Activity - Exercise:	Duration	Calories	Intensity

Other Notes, Vitamins, Supplements Meds:

_____

_____

_____

_____

	Calories	Carbs (g)	Sugars (g)	Fiber (g)	Protein (g)	Fat (g)
Date: _____						
Weight: _____						
Daily Goal: _____						
Breakfast: Time:						
Lunch: Time:						
Dinner: Time:						
Page Totals:						

	Calories	Carbs (g)	Sugars (g)	Fiber (g)	Protein (g)	Fat (g)
Sleep: _____ Water: _____ Mood: _____						
Other Meals / Snacks:						
Page Totals:						

Blood Sugar Log:	Before	After	Insulin	Meds
Breakfast				
Lunch				
Dinner				

Activity - Exercise:	Duration	Calories	Intensity

Other Notes, Vitamins, Supplements Meds:

_____

_____

_____

_____

	Calories	Carbs (g)	Sugars (g)	Fiber (g)	Protein (g)	Fat (g)
Date:						
Weight:						
Daily Goal:						
Breakfast: Time:						
Lunch: Time:						
Dinner: Time:						
Page Totals:						

	Calories	Carbs (g)	Sugars (g)	Fiber (g)	Protein (g)	Fat (g)
Sleep: _____						
Water: _____						
Mood: _____						
Other Meals / Snacks:						
Page Totals:						

Blood Sugar Log:	Before	After	Insulin	Meds
Breakfast				
Lunch				
Dinner				

Activity - Exercise:	Duration	Calories	Intensity

Other Notes, Vitamins, Supplements Meds:

_____

_____

_____

_____

	Calories	Carbs (g)	Sugars (g)	Fiber (g)	Protein (g)	Fat (g)
Date:						
Weight:						
Daily Goal:						
Breakfast: Time:						
Lunch: Time:						
Dinner: Time:						
Page Totals:						

		Calories	Carbs (g)	Sugars (g)	Fiber (g)	Protein (g)	Fat (g)
Sleep: _____							
Water: _____							
Mood: _____							
Other Meals / Snacks:							
Page Totals:							

Blood Sugar Log:	Before	After	Insulin	Meds
Breakfast				
Lunch				
Dinner				

Activity - Exercise:	Duration	Calories	Intensity

Other Notes, Vitamins, Supplements Meds:

_____

_____

_____

_____

	Calories	Carbs (g)	Sugars (g)	Fiber (g)	Protein (g)	Fat (g)
Date:						
Weight:						
Daily Goal:						
Breakfast: Time:						
Lunch: Time:						
Dinner: Time:						
Page Totals:						

	Calories	Carbs (g)	Sugars (g)	Fiber (g)	Protein (g)	Fat (g)
Sleep: _____						
Water: _____						
Mood: _____						
Other Meals / Snacks:						
Page Totals:						

Blood Sugar Log:	Before	After	Insulin	Meds
Breakfast				
Lunch				
Dinner				

Activity - Exercise:	Duration	Calories	Intensity

Other Notes, Vitamins, Supplements Meds:

_____

_____

_____

_____

	Calories	Carbs (g)	Sugars (g)	Fiber (g)	Protein (g)	Fat (g)
Date:						
Weight:						
Daily Goal:						
Breakfast: Time:						
Lunch: Time:						
Dinner: Time:						
Page Totals:						

	Calories	Carbs (g)	Sugars (g)	Fiber (g)	Protein (g)	Fat (g)
Sleep: _____ Water: _____ Mood: _____						
Other Meals / Snacks:						
Page Totals:						

Blood Sugar Log:	Before	After	Insulin	Meds
Breakfast				
Lunch				
Dinner				

Activity - Exercise:	Duration	Calories	Intensity

Other Notes, Vitamins, Supplements Meds:

_____

_____

_____

_____

	Calories	Carbs (g)	Sugars (g)	Fiber (g)	Protein (g)	Fat (g)
Date: _____						
Weight: _____						
Daily Goal: _____						
Breakfast: **Time:**						
Lunch: **Time:**						
Dinner: **Time:**						
Page Totals:						

		Calories	Carbs (g)	Sugars (g)	Fiber (g)	Protein (g)	Fat (g)
Sleep: _____							
Water: _____							
Mood: _____							

Other Meals / Snacks:	Calories	Carbs (g)	Sugars (g)	Fiber (g)	Protein (g)	Fat (g)
Page Totals:						

Blood Sugar Log:	Before	After	Insulin	Meds
Breakfast				
Lunch				
Dinner				

Activity - Exercise:	Duration	Calories	Intensity

Other Notes, Vitamins, Supplements Meds:

_____

_____

_____

_____

	Calories	Carbs (g)	Sugars (g)	Fiber (g)	Protein (g)	Fat (g)
Date: _____ Weight: _____ Daily Goal: _____						
Breakfast: Time:						
Lunch: Time:						
Dinner: Time:						
Page Totals:						

	Calories	Carbs (g)	Sugars (g)	Fiber (g)	Protein (g)	Fat (g)
Sleep: _____						
Water: _____						
Mood: _____						
Other Meals / Snacks:						
Page Totals:						

Blood Sugar Log:	Before	After	Insulin	Meds
Breakfast				
Lunch				
Dinner				

Activity - Exercise:	Duration	Calories	Intensity

Other Notes, Vitamins, Supplements Meds:

_____

_____

_____

_____

	Calories	Carbs (g)	Sugars (g)	Fiber (g)	Protein (g)	Fat (g)
Date:						
Weight:						
Daily Goal:						
Breakfast: Time:						
Lunch: Time:						
Dinner: Time:						
Page Totals:						

	Calories	Carbs (g)	Sugars (g)	Fiber (g)	Protein (g)	Fat (g)
Sleep: _____						
Water: _____						
Mood: _____						
Other Meals / Snacks:						
Page Totals:						

Blood Sugar Log:	Before	After	Insulin	Meds
Breakfast				
Lunch				
Dinner				

Activity - Exercise:	Duration	Calories	Intensity

Other Notes, Vitamins, Supplements Meds:

_____

_____

_____

_____

	Calories	Carbs (g)	Sugars (g)	Fiber (g)	Protein (g)	Fat (g)
Date: _____ Weight: _____ Daily Goal: _____						
Breakfast: Time:						
Lunch: Time:						
Dinner: Time:						
Page Totals:						

	Calories	Carbs (g)	Sugars (g)	Fiber (g)	Protein (g)	Fat (g)
Sleep: _____ Water: _____ Mood: _____						
Other Meals / Snacks:						
Page Totals:						

Blood Sugar Log:	Before	After	Insulin	Meds
Breakfast				
Lunch				
Dinner				

Activity - Exercise:	Duration	Calories	Intensity

Other Notes, Vitamins, Supplements Meds:

_____

_____

_____

_____

	Calories	Carbs (g)	Sugars (g)	Fiber (g)	Protein (g)	Fat (g)
Date: _____						
Weight: _____						
Daily Goal: _____						
Breakfast: Time:						
Lunch: Time:						
Dinner: Time:						
Page Totals:						

	Calories	Carbs (g)	Sugars (g)	Fiber (g)	Protein (g)	Fat (g)
Sleep: _____ Water: _____ Mood: _____						
Other Meals / Snacks:						
Page Totals:						

Blood Sugar Log:	Before	After	Insulin	Meds
Breakfast				
Lunch				
Dinner				

Activity - Exercise:	Duration	Calories	Intensity

Other Notes, Vitamins, Supplements Meds:

_____

_____

_____

_____

	Calories	Carbs (g)	Sugars (g)	Fiber (g)	Protein (g)	Fat (g)
Date: _____						
Weight: _____						
Daily Goal: _____						
Breakfast: Time:						
Lunch: Time:						
Dinner: Time:						
Page Totals:						

	Calories	Carbs (g)	Sugars (g)	Fiber (g)	Protein (g)	Fat (g)
Sleep: _____						
Water: _____						
Mood: _____						
Other Meals / Snacks:						
Page Totals:						

Blood Sugar Log:	Before	After	Insulin	Meds
Breakfast				
Lunch				
Dinner				

Activity - Exercise:	Duration	Calories	Intensity

Other Notes, Vitamins, Supplements Meds:

_____

_____

_____

_____

	Calories	Carbs (g)	Sugars (g)	Fiber (g)	Protein (g)	Fat (g)
Date: _____						
Weight: _____						
Daily Goal: _____						
Breakfast: Time:						
Lunch: Time:						
Dinner: Time:						
Page Totals:						

Sleep: _____

Water: _____

Mood: _____

	Calories	Carbs (g)	Sugars (g)	Fiber (g)	Protein (g)	Fat (g)
Other Meals / Snacks:						
Page Totals:						

Blood Sugar Log:	Before	After	Insulin	Meds
Breakfast				
Lunch				
Dinner				

Activity - Exercise:	Duration	Calories	Intensity

Other Notes, Vitamins, Supplements Meds:

_____

_____

_____

_____

	Calories	Carbs (g)	Sugars (g)	Fiber (g)	Protein (g)	Fat (g)
Date: _____						
Weight: _____						
Daily Goal: _____						
Breakfast: Time:						
Lunch: Time:						
Dinner: Time:						
Page Totals:						

	Calories	Carbs (g)	Sugars (g)	Fiber (g)	Protein (g)	Fat (g)
Sleep: _____ Water: _____ Mood: _____						
Other Meals / Snacks:						
Page Totals:						

Blood Sugar Log:	Before	After	Insulin	Meds
Breakfast				
Lunch				
Dinner				

Activity - Exercise:	Duration	Calories	Intensity

Other Notes, Vitamins, Supplements Meds:

_____

_____

_____

_____

	Calories	Carbs (g)	Sugars (g)	Fiber (g)	Protein (g)	Fat (g)
Date: _____						
Weight: _____						
Daily Goal: _____						
Breakfast: Time:						
Lunch: Time:						
Dinner: Time:						
Page Totals:						

		Calories	Carbs (g)	Sugars (g)	Fiber (g)	Protein (g)	Fat (g)
Sleep: _____							
Water: _____							
Mood: _____							
Other Meals / Snacks:							
Page Totals:							

Blood Sugar Log:	Before	After	Insulin	Meds
Breakfast				
Lunch				
Dinner				

Activity - Exercise:	Duration	Calories	Intensity

Other Notes, Vitamins, Supplements Meds:

_____

_____

_____

_____

	Calories	Carbs (g)	Sugars (g)	Fiber (g)	Protein (g)	Fat (g)
Date: _____						
Weight: _____						
Daily Goal: _____						
Breakfast: Time:						
Lunch: Time:						
Dinner: Time:						
Page Totals:						

Sleep:		Calories	Carbs (g)	Sugars (g)	Fiber (g)	Protein (g)	Fat (g)
Water:							
Mood:							
Other Meals / Snacks:							
Page Totals:							

Blood Sugar Log:	Before	After	Insulin	Meds
Breakfast				
Lunch				
Dinner				

Activity - Exercise:	Duration	Calories	Intensity

Other Notes, Vitamins, Supplements Meds:

_____

_____

_____

_____

	Calories	Carbs (g)	Sugars (g)	Fiber (g)	Protein (g)	Fat (g)
Date: _____						
Weight: _____						
Daily Goal: _____						
Breakfast: Time:						
Lunch: Time:						
Dinner: Time:						
Page Totals:						

	Calories	Carbs (g)	Sugars (g)	Fiber (g)	Protein (g)	Fat (g)
Sleep: _____ Water: _____ Mood: _____						
Other Meals / Snacks:						
Page Totals:						

Blood Sugar Log:	Before	After	Insulin	Meds
Breakfast				
Lunch				
Dinner				

Activity - Exercise:	Duration	Calories	Intensity

Other Notes, Vitamins, Supplements Meds:

_____

_____

_____

_____

	Calories	Carbs (g)	Sugars (g)	Fiber (g)	Protein (g)	Fat (g)
Date:						
Weight:						
Daily Goal:						
Breakfast: Time:						
Lunch: Time:						
Dinner: Time:						
Page Totals:						

	Calories	Carbs (g)	Sugars (g)	Fiber (g)	Protein (g)	Fat (g)
Sleep: _____ Water: _____ Mood: _____						
Other Meals / Snacks:						
Page Totals:						

Blood Sugar Log:	Before	After	Insulin	Meds
Breakfast				
Lunch				
Dinner				

Activity - Exercise:	Duration	Calories	Intensity

Other Notes, Vitamins, Supplements Meds:

_____

_____

_____

_____

	Calories	Carbs (g)	Sugars (g)	Fiber (g)	Protein (g)	Fat (g)
Date: _____						
Weight: _____						
Daily Goal: _____						
Breakfast: Time:						
Lunch: Time:						
Dinner: Time:						
Page Totals:						

Sleep: _____	Calories	Carbs (g)	Sugars (g)	Fiber (g)	Protein (g)	Fat (g)
Water: _____						
Mood: _____						
Other Meals / Snacks:						
Page Totals:						

Blood Sugar Log:	Before	After	Insulin	Meds
Breakfast				
Lunch				
Dinner				

Activity - Exercise:	Duration	Calories	Intensity

Other Notes, Vitamins, Supplements Meds:

_____

_____

_____

_____

	Calories	Carbs (g)	Sugars (g)	Fiber (g)	Protein (g)	Fat (g)
Date: _____						
Weight: _____						
Daily Goal: _____						
Breakfast: Time:						
Lunch: Time:						
Dinner: Time:						
Page Totals:						

Sleep:		Calories	Carbs (g)	Sugars (g)	Fiber (g)	Protein (g)	Fat (g)
Water:							
Mood:							
Other Meals / Snacks:							
Page Totals:							

Blood Sugar Log:	Before	After	Insulin	Meds
Breakfast				
Lunch				
Dinner				

Activity - Exercise:	Duration	Calories	Intensity

Other Notes, Vitamins, Supplements Meds:

_____

_____

_____

_____

	Calories	Carbs (g)	Sugars (g)	Fiber (g)	Protein (g)	Fat (g)
Date: _____						
Weight: _____						
Daily Goal: _____						
Breakfast: Time:						
Lunch: Time:						
Dinner: Time:						
Page Totals:						

	Calories	Carbs (g)	Sugars (g)	Fiber (g)	Protein (g)	Fat (g)
Sleep: _____ Water: _____ Mood: _____						
Other Meals / Snacks:						
Page Totals:						

Blood Sugar Log:	Before	After	Insulin	Meds
Breakfast				
Lunch				
Dinner				

Activity - Exercise:	Duration	Calories	Intensity

Other Notes, Vitamins, Supplements Meds:

_____

_____

_____

_____

	Calories	Carbs (g)	Sugars (g)	Fiber (g)	Protein (g)	Fat (g)
Date:						
Weight:						
Daily Goal:						
Breakfast: Time:						
Lunch: Time:						
Dinner: Time:						
Page Totals:						

	Calories	Carbs (g)	Sugars (g)	Fiber (g)	Protein (g)	Fat (g)
Sleep: _____ Water: _____ Mood: _____						
Other Meals / Snacks:						
Page Totals:						

Blood Sugar Log:	Before	After	Insulin	Meds
Breakfast				
Lunch				
Dinner				

Activity - Exercise:	Duration	Calories	Intensity

Other Notes, Vitamins, Supplements Meds:

_____

_____

_____

_____

	Calories	Carbs (g)	Sugars (g)	Fiber (g)	Protein (g)	Fat (g)
Date: _____						
Weight: _____						
Daily Goal: _____						
Breakfast: Time:						
Lunch: Time:						
Dinner: Time:						
Page Totals:						

	Calories	Carbs (g)	Sugars (g)	Fiber (g)	Protein (g)	Fat (g)
Sleep: _____ Water: _____ Mood: _____						

Other Meals / Snacks:						
Page Totals:						

Blood Sugar Log:	Before	After	Insulin	Meds
Breakfast				
Lunch				
Dinner				

Activity - Exercise:	Duration	Calories	Intensity

Other Notes, Vitamins, Supplements Meds:

_____

_____

_____

_____

	Calories	Carbs (g)	Sugars (g)	Fiber (g)	Protein (g)	Fat (g)
Date: _____ Weight: _____ Daily Goal: _____						
Breakfast: Time:						
Lunch: Time:						
Dinner: Time:						
Page Totals:						

		Calories	Carbs (g)	Sugars (g)	Fiber (g)	Protein (g)	Fat (g)
Sleep: _____							
Water: _____							
Mood: _____							
Other Meals / Snacks:							
Page Totals:							

Blood Sugar Log:	Before	After	Insulin	Meds
Breakfast				
Lunch				
Dinner				

Activity - Exercise:	Duration	Calories	Intensity

Other Notes, Vitamins, Supplements Meds:

_____
_____
_____
_____

	Calories	Carbs (g)	Sugars (g)	Fiber (g)	Protein (g)	Fat (g)
Date:						
Weight:						
Daily Goal:						
Breakfast:				Time:		
Lunch:				Time:		
Dinner:				Time:		
Page Totals:						

	Calories	Carbs (g)	Sugars (g)	Fiber (g)	Protein (g)	Fat (g)
Sleep: _____ Water: _____ Mood: _____						
Other Meals / Snacks:						
Page Totals:						

Blood Sugar Log:	Before	After	Insulin	Meds
Breakfast				
Lunch				
Dinner				

Activity - Exercise:	Duration	Calories	Intensity

Other Notes, Vitamins, Supplements Meds:

_____

_____

_____

_____

	Calories	Carbs (g)	Sugars (g)	Fiber (g)	Protein (g)	Fat (g)
Date:						
Weight:						
Daily Goal:						
Breakfast:				Time:		
Lunch:				Time:		
Dinner:				Time:		
Page Totals:						

	Calories	Carbs (g)	Sugars (g)	Fiber (g)	Protein (g)	Fat (g)
Sleep: _____ Water: _____ Mood: _____						
Other Meals / Snacks:						
Page Totals:						

Blood Sugar Log:	Before	After	Insulin	Meds
Breakfast				
Lunch				
Dinner				

Activity - Exercise:	Duration	Calories	Intensity

Other Notes, Vitamins, Supplements Meds:

_____

_____

_____

_____

	Calories	Carbs (g)	Sugars (g)	Fiber (g)	Protein (g)	Fat (g)
Date: _____						
Weight: _____						
Daily Goal: _____						
Breakfast: Time:						
Lunch: Time:						
Dinner: Time:						
Page Totals:						

Sleep: _____	Calories	Carbs (g)	Sugars (g)	Fiber (g)	Protein (g)	Fat (g)
Water: _____						
Mood: _____						

Other Meals / Snacks:	Calories	Carbs (g)	Sugars (g)	Fiber (g)	Protein (g)	Fat (g)
Page Totals:						

Blood Sugar Log:	Before	After	Insulin	Meds
Breakfast				
Lunch				
Dinner				

Activity - Exercise:	Duration	Calories	Intensity

Other Notes, Vitamins, Supplements Meds:

_____

_____

_____

_____

	Calories	Carbs (g)	Sugars (g)	Fiber (g)	Protein (g)	Fat (g)
Date: _____ Weight: _____ Daily Goal: _____						
Breakfast: Time:						
Lunch: Time:						
Dinner: Time:						
Page Totals:						

	Calories	Carbs (g)	Sugars (g)	Fiber (g)	Protein (g)	Fat (g)
Sleep: _____						
Water: _____						
Mood: _____						
Other Meals / Snacks:						
Page Totals:						

Blood Sugar Log:	Before	After	Insulin	Meds
Breakfast				
Lunch				
Dinner				

Activity - Exercise:	Duration	Calories	Intensity

Other Notes, Vitamins, Supplements Meds:

_____

_____

_____

_____

	Calories	Carbs (g)	Sugars (g)	Fiber (g)	Protein (g)	Fat (g)
Date: _____						
Weight: _____						
Daily Goal: _____						
Breakfast: Time:						
Lunch: Time:						
Dinner: Time:						
Page Totals:						

	Calories	Carbs (g)	Sugars (g)	Fiber (g)	Protein (g)	Fat (g)
Sleep: _____ Water: _____ Mood: _____						
Other Meals / Snacks:						
Page Totals:						

Blood Sugar Log:	Before	After	Insulin	Meds
Breakfast				
Lunch				
Dinner				

Activity - Exercise:	Duration	Calories	Intensity

Other Notes, Vitamins, Supplements Meds:

_____

_____

_____

_____

	Calories	Carbs (g)	Sugars (g)	Fiber (g)	Protein (g)	Fat (g)
Date: _____						
Weight: _____						
Daily Goal: _____						
Breakfast: Time:						
Lunch: Time:						
Dinner: Time:						
Page Totals:						

		Calories	Carbs (g)	Sugars (g)	Fiber (g)	Protein (g)	Fat (g)
Sleep: _____							
Water: _____							
Mood: _____							
Other Meals / Snacks:							
Page Totals:							

Blood Sugar Log:	Before	After	Insulin	Meds
Breakfast				
Lunch				
Dinner				

Activity - Exercise:	Duration	Calories	Intensity

Other Notes, Vitamins, Supplements Meds:

_____

_____

_____

_____

	Calories	Carbs (g)	Sugars (g)	Fiber (g)	Protein (g)	Fat (g)
Date:						
Weight:						
Daily Goal:						
Breakfast: Time:						
Lunch: Time:						
Dinner: Time:						
Page Totals:						

	Calories	Carbs (g)	Sugars (g)	Fiber (g)	Protein (g)	Fat (g)
Sleep: _____ Water: _____ Mood: _____						
Other Meals / Snacks:						
Page Totals:						

Blood Sugar Log:	Before	After	Insulin	Meds
Breakfast				
Lunch				
Dinner				

Activity - Exercise:	Duration	Calories	Intensity

Other Notes, Vitamins, Supplements Meds:

_____

_____

_____

_____

	Calories	Carbs (g)	Sugars (g)	Fiber (g)	Protein (g)	Fat (g)
Date: _____ Weight: _____ Daily Goal: _____						
Breakfast: Time:						
Lunch: Time:						
Dinner: Time:						
Page Totals:						

	Calories	Carbs (g)	Sugars (g)	Fiber (g)	Protein (g)	Fat (g)
Sleep: _____ Water: _____ Mood: _____						
Other Meals / Snacks:						
Page Totals:						

Blood Sugar Log:	Before	After	Insulin	Meds
Breakfast				
Lunch				
Dinner				

Activity - Exercise:	Duration	Calories	Intensity

Other Notes, Vitamins, Supplements Meds:

_____

_____

_____

_____

	Calories	Carbs (g)	Sugars (g)	Fiber (g)	Protein (g)	Fat (g)
Date:						
Weight:						
Daily Goal:						
Breakfast:				Time:		
Lunch:				Time:		
Dinner:				Time:		
Page Totals:						

	Calories	Carbs (g)	Sugars (g)	Fiber (g)	Protein (g)	Fat (g)
Sleep: _____						
Water: _____						
Mood: _____						
Other Meals / Snacks:						
Page Totals:						

Blood Sugar Log:	Before	After	Insulin	Meds
Breakfast				
Lunch				
Dinner				

Activity - Exercise:	Duration	Calories	Intensity

Other Notes, Vitamins, Supplements Meds:

_____

_____

_____

_____

	Calories	Carbs (g)	Sugars (g)	Fiber (g)	Protein (g)	Fat (g)
Date: _____						
Weight: _____						
Daily Goal: _____						
Breakfast: Time:						
Lunch: Time:						
Dinner: Time:						
Page Totals:						

	Calories	Carbs (g)	Sugars (g)	Fiber (g)	Protein (g)	Fat (g)
Sleep: _____ Water: _____ Mood: _____						
Other Meals / Snacks:						
Page Totals:						

Blood Sugar Log:	Before	After	Insulin	Meds
Breakfast				
Lunch				
Dinner				

Activity - Exercise:	Duration	Calories	Intensity

Other Notes, Vitamins, Supplements Meds:

_____

_____

_____

_____

	Calories	Carbs (g)	Sugars (g)	Fiber (g)	Protein (g)	Fat (g)
Date: _____						
Weight: _____						
Daily Goal: _____						
Breakfast: Time:						
Lunch: Time:						
Dinner: Time:						
Page Totals:						

	Calories	Carbs (g)	Sugars (g)	Fiber (g)	Protein (g)	Fat (g)
Sleep: _____ Water: _____ Mood: _____						
Other Meals / Snacks:						
Page Totals:						

Blood Sugar Log:	Before	After	Insulin	Meds
Breakfast				
Lunch				
Dinner				

Activity - Exercise:	Duration	Calories	Intensity

Other Notes, Vitamins, Supplements Meds:

_____

_____

_____

_____

	Calories	Carbs (g)	Sugars (g)	Fiber (g)	Protein (g)	Fat (g)
Date: _____						
Weight: _____						
Daily Goal: _____						
Breakfast: Time:						
Lunch: Time:						
Dinner: Time:						
Page Totals:						

	Calories	Carbs (g)	Sugars (g)	Fiber (g)	Protein (g)	Fat (g)
Sleep: _____						
Water: _____						
Mood: _____						
Other Meals / Snacks:						
Page Totals:						

Blood Sugar Log:	Before	After	Insulin	Meds
Breakfast				
Lunch				
Dinner				

Activity - Exercise:	Duration	Calories	Intensity

Other Notes, Vitamins, Supplements Meds:

_____

_____

_____

_____

	Calories	Carbs (g)	Sugars (g)	Fiber (g)	Protein (g)	Fat (g)
Date: _____						
Weight: _____						
Daily Goal: _____						
Breakfast: Time:						
Lunch: Time:						
Dinner: Time:						
Page Totals:						

		Calories	Carbs (g)	Sugars (g)	Fiber (g)	Protein (g)	Fat (g)
Sleep: _____							
Water: _____							
Mood: _____							
Other Meals / Snacks:							
Page Totals:							

Blood Sugar Log:	Before	After	Insulin	Meds
Breakfast				
Lunch				
Dinner				

Activity - Exercise:	Duration	Calories	Intensity

Other Notes, Vitamins, Supplements Meds:

_____

_____

_____

_____

	Calories	Carbs (g)	Sugars (g)	Fiber (g)	Protein (g)	Fat (g)
Date: _____						
Weight: _____						
Daily Goal: _____						
Breakfast: Time:						
Lunch: Time:						
Dinner: Time:						
Page Totals:						

		Calories	Carbs (g)	Sugars (g)	Fiber (g)	Protein (g)	Fat (g)
Sleep: _____							
Water: _____							
Mood: _____							
Other Meals / Snacks:							
Page Totals:							

Blood Sugar Log:	Before	After	Insulin	Meds
Breakfast				
Lunch				
Dinner				

Activity - Exercise:	Duration	Calories	Intensity

Other Notes, Vitamins, Supplements Meds:

_____

_____

_____

_____

	Calories	Carbs (g)	Sugars (g)	Fiber (g)	Protein (g)	Fat (g)
Date: _____						
Weight: _____						
Daily Goal: _____						
Breakfast: Time:						
Lunch: Time:						
Dinner: Time:						
Page Totals:						

	Calories	Carbs (g)	Sugars (g)	Fiber (g)	Protein (g)	Fat (g)
Sleep: _____ Water: _____ Mood: _____						
Other Meals / Snacks:						
Page Totals:						

Blood Sugar Log:	Before	After	Insulin	Meds
Breakfast				
Lunch				
Dinner				

Activity - Exercise:	Duration	Calories	Intensity

Other Notes, Vitamins, Supplements Meds:

_____

_____

_____

_____

	Calories	Carbs (g)	Sugars (g)	Fiber (g)	Protein (g)	Fat (g)
Date: _____						
Weight: _____						
Daily Goal: _____						
Breakfast: Time:						
Lunch: Time:						
Dinner: Time:						
Page Totals:						

Sleep: _____ Water: _____ Mood: _____	Calories	Carbs (g)	Sugars (g)	Fiber (g)	Protein (g)	Fat (g)
Other Meals / Snacks:						
Page Totals:						

Blood Sugar Log:	Before	After	Insulin	Meds
Breakfast				
Lunch				
Dinner				

Activity - Exercise:	Duration	Calories	Intensity

Other Notes, Vitamins, Supplements Meds:

_____

_____

_____

_____

	Calories	Carbs (g)	Sugars (g)	Fiber (g)	Protein (g)	Fat (g)
Date: _____						
Weight: _____						
Daily Goal: _____						
Breakfast: Time:						
Lunch: Time:						
Dinner: Time:						
Page Totals:						

		Calories	Carbs (g)	Sugars (g)	Fiber (g)	Protein (g)	Fat (g)
Sleep: _____							
Water: _____							
Mood: _____							
Other Meals / Snacks:							
Page Totals:							

Blood Sugar Log:	Before	After	Insulin	Meds
Breakfast				
Lunch				
Dinner				

Activity - Exercise:	Duration	Calories	Intensity

Other Notes, Vitamins, Supplements Meds:

_____

_____

_____

_____

	Calories	Carbs (g)	Sugars (g)	Fiber (g)	Protein (g)	Fat (g)
Date:						
Weight:						
Daily Goal:						
Breakfast: Time:						
Lunch: Time:						
Dinner: Time:						
Page Totals:						

	Calories	Carbs (g)	Sugars (g)	Fiber (g)	Protein (g)	Fat (g)
Sleep: _____ Water: _____ Mood: _____						
Other Meals / Snacks:						
Page Totals:						

Blood Sugar Log:	Before	After	Insulin	Meds
Breakfast				
Lunch				
Dinner				

Activity - Exercise:	Duration	Calories	Intensity

Other Notes, Vitamins, Supplements Meds:

_____

_____

_____

_____

	Calories	Carbs (g)	Sugars (g)	Fiber (g)	Protein (g)	Fat (g)
Date: _____						
Weight: _____						
Daily Goal: _____						
Breakfast: Time:						
Lunch: Time:						
Dinner: Time:						
Page Totals:						

	Calories	Carbs (g)	Sugars (g)	Fiber (g)	Protein (g)	Fat (g)
Sleep: _____ Water: _____ Mood: _____						
Other Meals / Snacks:						
Page Totals:						

Blood Sugar Log:	Before	After	Insulin	Meds
Breakfast				
Lunch				
Dinner				

Activity - Exercise:	Duration	Calories	Intensity

Other Notes, Vitamins, Supplements Meds:

_____

_____

_____

_____

	Calories	Carbs (g)	Sugars (g)	Fiber (g)	Protein (g)	Fat (g)
Date: _____						
Weight: _____						
Daily Goal: _____						
Breakfast: Time:						
Lunch: Time:						
Dinner: Time:						
Page Totals:						

Sleep: _____	Calories	Carbs (g)	Sugars (g)	Fiber (g)	Protein (g)	Fat (g)
Water: _____						
Mood: _____						
Other Meals / Snacks:						
Page Totals:						

Blood Sugar Log:	Before	After	Insulin	Meds
Breakfast				
Lunch				
Dinner				

Activity - Exercise:	Duration	Calories	Intensity

Other Notes, Vitamins, Supplements Meds:

_____

_____

_____

_____

	Calories	Carbs (g)	Sugars (g)	Fiber (g)	Protein (g)	Fat (g)
Date: _____						
Weight: _____						
Daily Goal: _____						
Breakfast: Time:						
Lunch: Time:						
Dinner: Time:						
Page Totals:						

	Calories	Carbs (g)	Sugars (g)	Fiber (g)	Protein (g)	Fat (g)
Sleep: _____						
Water: _____						
Mood: _____						
Other Meals / Snacks:						
Page Totals:						

Blood Sugar Log:	Before	After	Insulin	Meds
Breakfast				
Lunch				
Dinner				

Activity - Exercise:	Duration	Calories	Intensity

Other Notes, Vitamins, Supplements Meds:

_____

_____

_____

_____

	Calories	Carbs (g)	Sugars (g)	Fiber (g)	Protein (g)	Fat (g)
Date:						
Weight:						
Daily Goal:						
Breakfast:				Time:		
Lunch:				Time:		
Dinner:				Time:		
Page Totals:						

	Calories	Carbs (g)	Sugars (g)	Fiber (g)	Protein (g)	Fat (g)
Sleep: _____						
Water: _____						
Mood: _____						
Other Meals / Snacks:						
Page Totals:						

Blood Sugar Log:	Before	After	Insulin	Meds
Breakfast				
Lunch				
Dinner				

Activity - Exercise:	Duration	Calories	Intensity

Other Notes, Vitamins, Supplements Meds:

_____

_____

_____

_____

	Calories	Carbs (g)	Sugars (g)	Fiber (g)	Protein (g)	Fat (g)
Date: _____						
Weight: _____						
Daily Goal: _____						
Breakfast: Time:						
Lunch: Time:						
Dinner: Time:						
Page Totals:						

Sleep: _____

Water: _____

Mood: _____

Other Meals / Snacks:	Calories	Carbs (g)	Sugars (g)	Fiber (g)	Protein (g)	Fat (g)
Page Totals:						

Blood Sugar Log:	Before	After	Insulin	Meds
Breakfast				
Lunch				
Dinner				

Activity - Exercise:	Duration	Calories	Intensity

Other Notes, Vitamins, Supplements Meds:

_____

_____

_____

_____

	Calories	Carbs (g)	Sugars (g)	Fiber (g)	Protein (g)	Fat (g)
Date: _____						
Weight: _____						
Daily Goal: _____						
Breakfast: Time:						
Lunch: Time:						
Dinner: Time:						
Page Totals:						

	Calories	Carbs (g)	Sugars (g)	Fiber (g)	Protein (g)	Fat (g)
Sleep: _____ Water: _____ Mood: _____						
Other Meals / Snacks:						
Page Totals:						

Blood Sugar Log:	Before	After	Insulin	Meds
Breakfast				
Lunch				
Dinner				

Activity - Exercise:	Duration	Calories	Intensity

Other Notes, Vitamins, Supplements Meds:

_____

_____

_____

_____

	Calories	Carbs (g)	Sugars (g)	Fiber (g)	Protein (g)	Fat (g)
Date:						
Weight:						
Daily Goal:						
Breakfast: Time:						
Lunch: Time:						
Dinner: Time:						
Page Totals:						

	Calories	Carbs (g)	Sugars (g)	Fiber (g)	Protein (g)	Fat (g)
Sleep: _____ Water: _____ Mood: _____						
Other Meals / Snacks:						
Page Totals:						

Blood Sugar Log:	Before	After	Insulin	Meds
Breakfast				
Lunch				
Dinner				

Activity - Exercise:	Duration	Calories	Intensity

Other Notes, Vitamins, Supplements Meds:

_____

_____

_____

_____

	Calories	Carbs (g)	Sugars (g)	Fiber (g)	Protein (g)	Fat (g)
Date:						
Weight:						
Daily Goal:						
Breakfast: Time:						
Lunch: Time:						
Dinner: Time:						
Page Totals:						

	Calories	Carbs (g)	Sugars (g)	Fiber (g)	Protein (g)	Fat (g)
Sleep: _____ Water: _____ Mood: _____						
Other Meals / Snacks:						
Page Totals:						

Blood Sugar Log:	Before	After	Insulin	Meds
Breakfast				
Lunch				
Dinner				

Activity - Exercise:	Duration	Calories	Intensity

Other Notes, Vitamins, Supplements Meds:

_____

_____

_____

_____

	Calories	Carbs (g)	Sugars (g)	Fiber (g)	Protein (g)	Fat (g)
Date: _____ Weight: _____ Daily Goal: _____						
Breakfast: Time:						
Lunch: Time:						
Dinner: Time:						
Page Totals:						

	Calories	Carbs (g)	Sugars (g)	Fiber (g)	Protein (g)	Fat (g)
Sleep: _____ Water: _____ Mood: _____						
Other Meals / Snacks:						
Page Totals:						

Blood Sugar Log:	Before	After	Insulin	Meds
Breakfast				
Lunch				
Dinner				

Activity - Exercise:	Duration	Calories	Intensity

Other Notes, Vitamins, Supplements Meds:

_____

_____

_____

_____

	Calories	Carbs (g)	Sugars (g)	Fiber (g)	Protein (g)	Fat (g)
Date:						
Weight:						
Daily Goal:						
Breakfast: Time:						
Lunch: Time:						
Dinner: Time:						
Page Totals:						

	Calories	Carbs (g)	Sugars (g)	Fiber (g)	Protein (g)	Fat (g)
Sleep: _____						
Water: _____						
Mood: _____						
Other Meals / Snacks:						
Page Totals:						

Blood Sugar Log:	Before	After	Insulin	Meds
Breakfast				
Lunch				
Dinner				

Activity - Exercise:	Duration	Calories	Intensity

Other Notes, Vitamins, Supplements Meds:

_____

_____

_____

_____

	Calories	Carbs (g)	Sugars (g)	Fiber (g)	Protein (g)	Fat (g)
Date:						
Weight:						
Daily Goal:						
Breakfast: Time:						
Lunch: Time:						
Dinner: Time:						
Page Totals:						

	Calories	Carbs (g)	Sugars (g)	Fiber (g)	Protein (g)	Fat (g)
Sleep: _____						
Water: _____						
Mood: _____						
Other Meals / Snacks:						
Page Totals:						

Blood Sugar Log:	Before	After	Insulin	Meds
Breakfast				
Lunch				
Dinner				

Activity - Exercise:	Duration	Calories	Intensity

Other Notes, Vitamins, Supplements Meds:

_____

_____

_____

_____

	Calories	Carbs (g)	Sugars (g)	Fiber (g)	Protein (g)	Fat (g)
Date: _____ Weight: _____ Daily Goal: _____						
Breakfast: Time:						
Lunch: Time:						
Dinner: Time:						
Page Totals:						

	Calories	Carbs (g)	Sugars (g)	Fiber (g)	Protein (g)	Fat (g)
Sleep: _____ Water: _____ Mood: _____						
Other Meals / Snacks:						
Page Totals:						

Blood Sugar Log:	Before	After	Insulin	Meds
Breakfast				
Lunch				
Dinner				

Activity - Exercise:	Duration	Calories	Intensity

Other Notes, Vitamins, Supplements Meds:

_____

_____

_____

_____

	Calories	Carbs (g)	Sugars (g)	Fiber (g)	Protein (g)	Fat (g)
Date:						
Weight:						
Daily Goal:						
Breakfast: Time:						
Lunch: Time:						
Dinner: Time:						
Page Totals:						

Sleep: _____

Water: _____

Mood: _____

Other Meals / Snacks:	Calories	Carbs (g)	Sugars (g)	Fiber (g)	Protein (g)	Fat (g)
Page Totals:						

Blood Sugar Log:	Before	After	Insulin	Meds
Breakfast				
Lunch				
Dinner				

Activity - Exercise:	Duration	Calories	Intensity

Other Notes, Vitamins, Supplements Meds:

_____

_____

_____

_____

	Calories	Carbs (g)	Sugars (g)	Fiber (g)	Protein (g)	Fat (g)
Date: _____						
Weight: _____						
Daily Goal: _____						
Breakfast: Time:						
Lunch: Time:						
Dinner: Time:						
Page Totals:						

	Calories	Carbs (g)	Sugars (g)	Fiber (g)	Protein (g)	Fat (g)
Sleep: _____						
Water: _____						
Mood: _____						
Other Meals / Snacks:						
Page Totals:						

Blood Sugar Log:	Before	After	Insulin	Meds
Breakfast				
Lunch				
Dinner				

Activity - Exercise:	Duration	Calories	Intensity

Other Notes, Vitamins, Supplements Meds:

_____

_____

_____

_____

	Calories	Carbs (g)	Sugars (g)	Fiber (g)	Protein (g)	Fat (g)
Date: _____						
Weight: _____						
Daily Goal: _____						
Breakfast: Time:						
Lunch: Time:						
Dinner: Time:						
Page Totals:						

Sleep: _____	Calories	Carbs (g)	Sugars (g)	Fiber (g)	Protein (g)	Fat (g)
Water: _____						
Mood: _____						
Other Meals / Snacks:						
Page Totals:						

Blood Sugar Log:	Before	After	Insulin	Meds
Breakfast				
Lunch				
Dinner				

Activity - Exercise:	Duration	Calories	Intensity

Other Notes, Vitamins, Supplements Meds:

_____

_____

_____

_____

Note:

Note:

Note:

Note:

Note:

Made in United States
North Haven, CT
08 May 2022

19021031R00072